I0435980

Water: The Coolest Drink Around

Water: The Coolest Drink Around
Written by Lynn Esmail
Illustrated by Patrick Eichhold

Copyright © 2016 Lynn Esmail and Patrick Eichhold
All rights reserved. This book or any portion thereof
may not be reproduced or used in any manner whatsoever
without the express written permission of the publisher
except for the use of brief quotations in a book review.

First Printing, 2016

ISBN 978-1-5323-0184-1

www.BedtimeStorybooksForHealth.com
contactus@bedtimestorybooksforhealth.com

Water

The Coolest Drink Around!

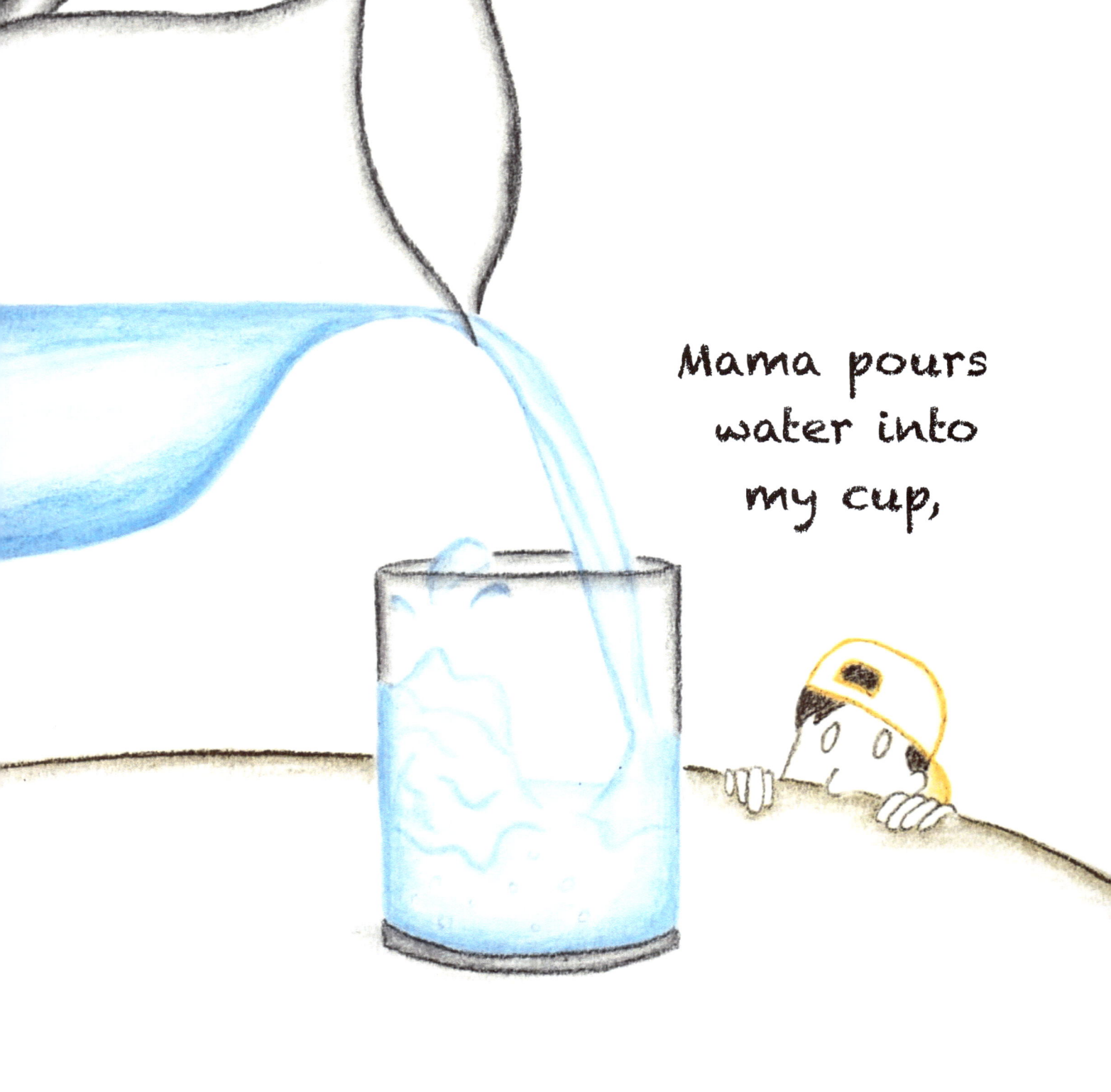

Mama pours water into my cup,

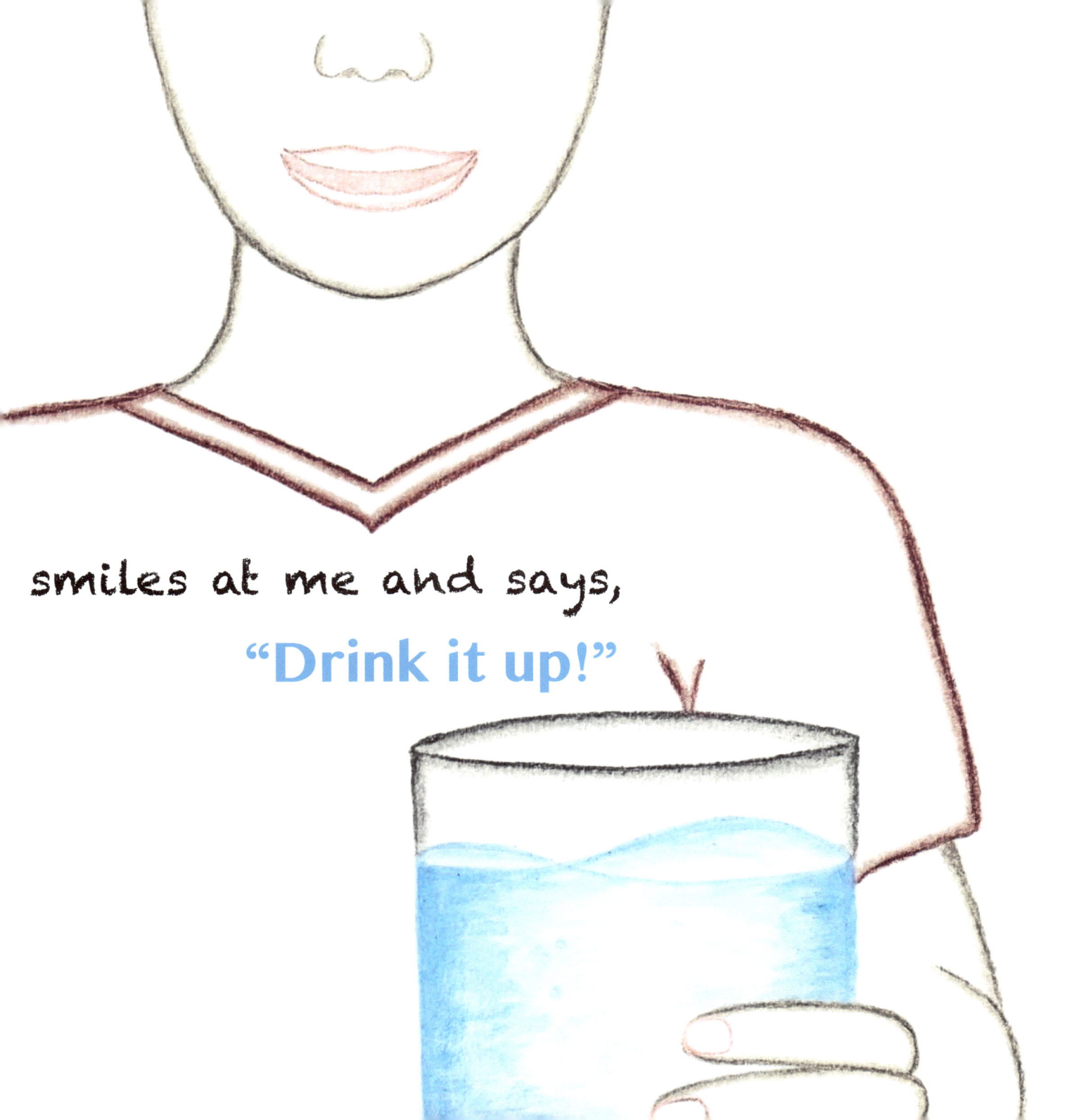

smiles at me and says,

"Drink it up!"

I feel so **strong** as I gulp it down,

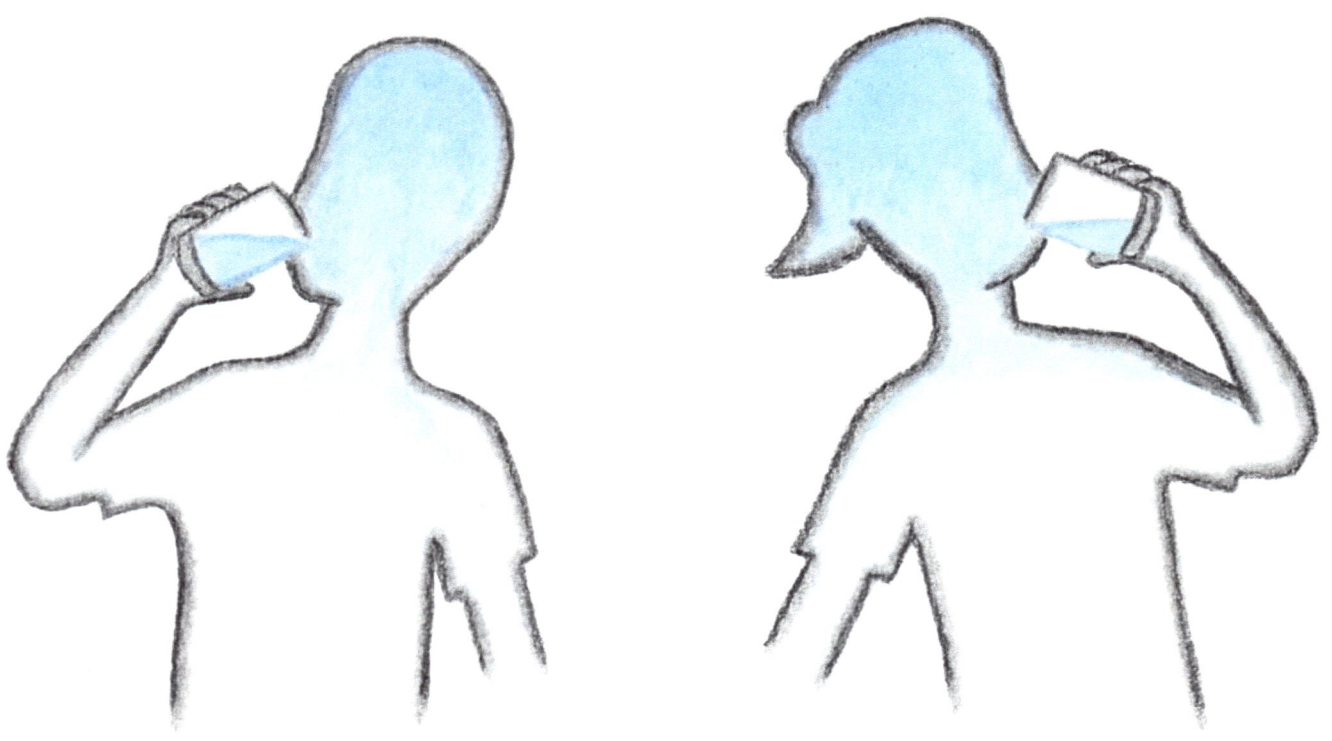

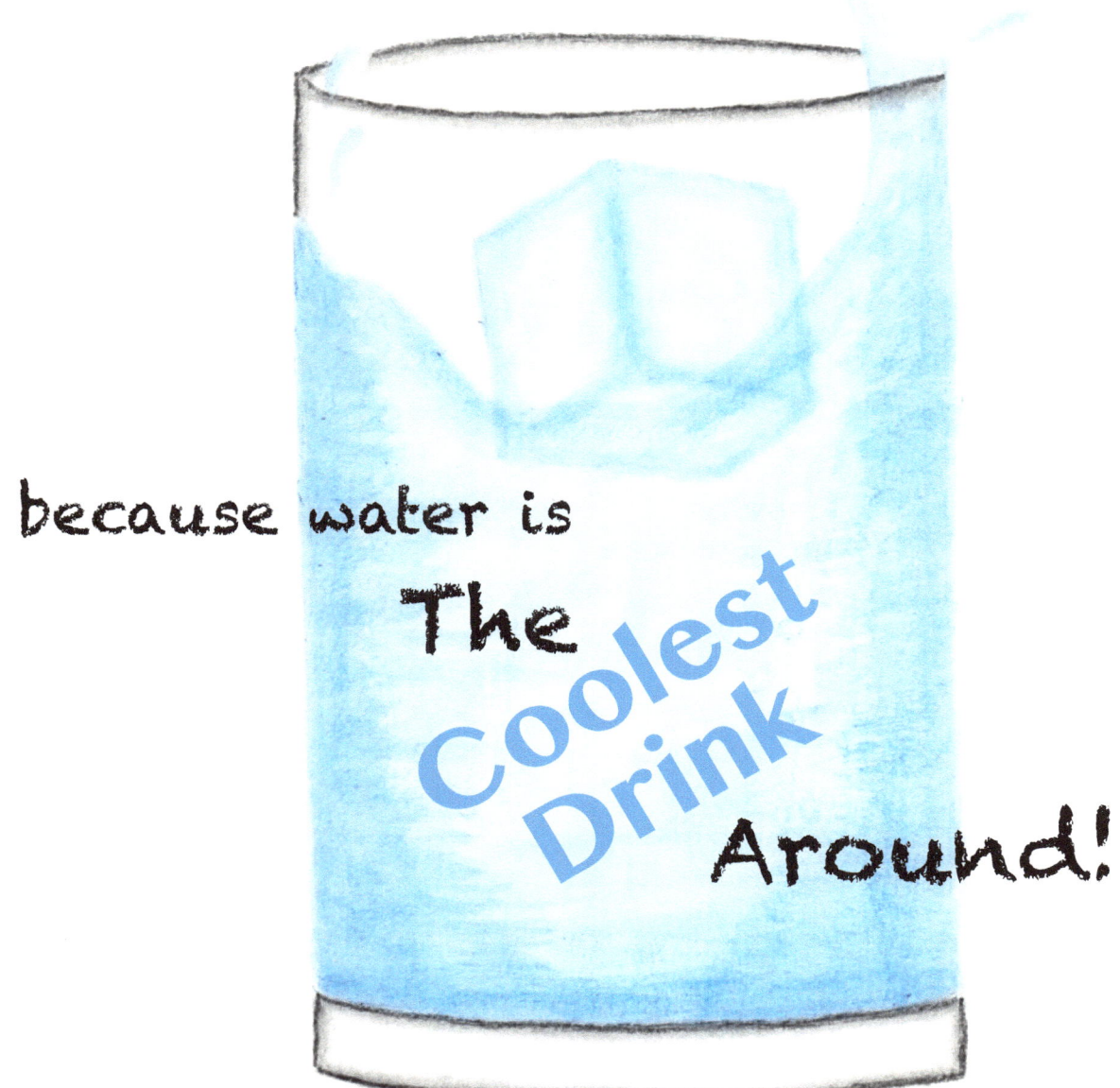

because water is

The

Coolest
Drink

Around!

When the cows come home
after being on the loose,

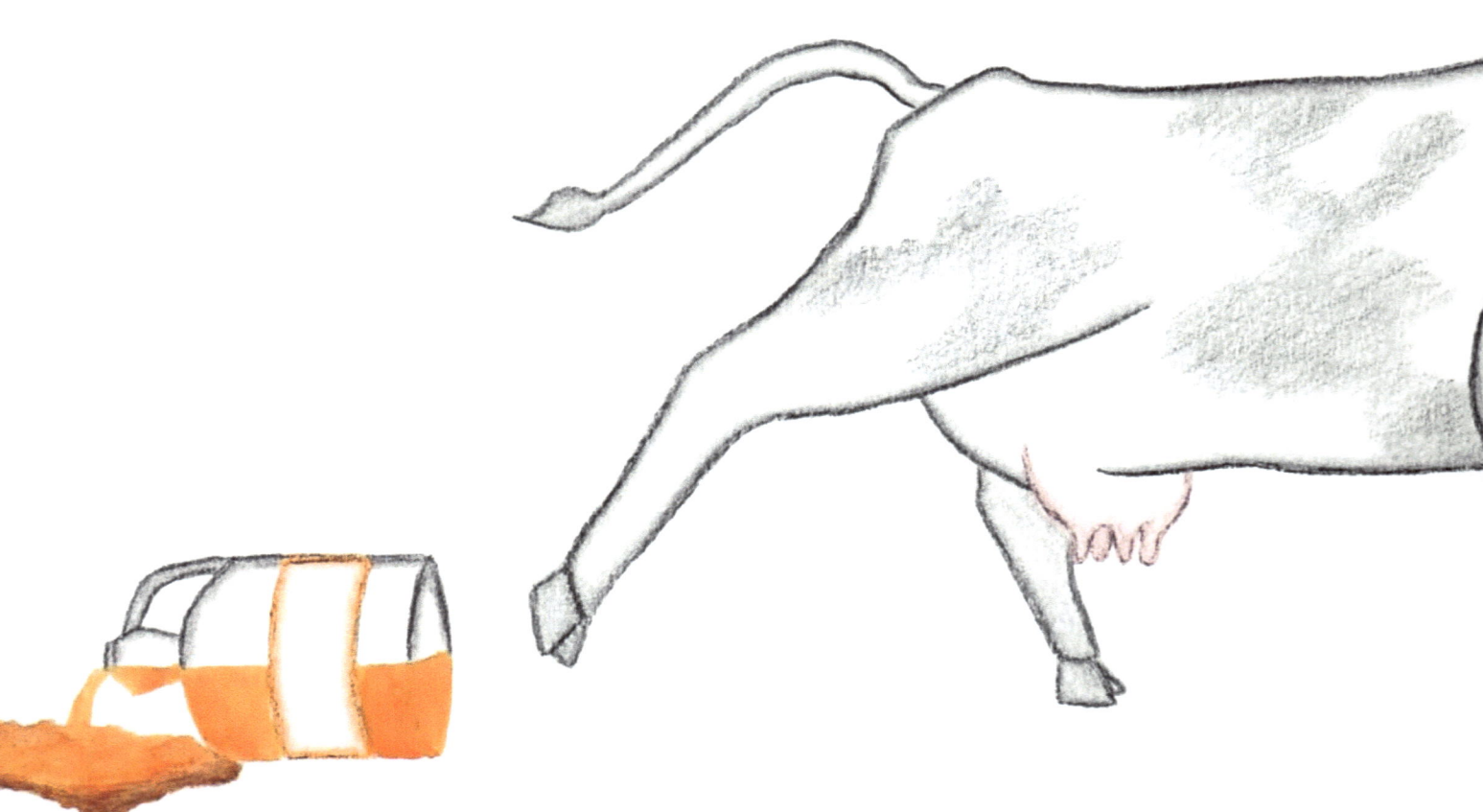

does the farmer fill their
trough with **sugary juice?**

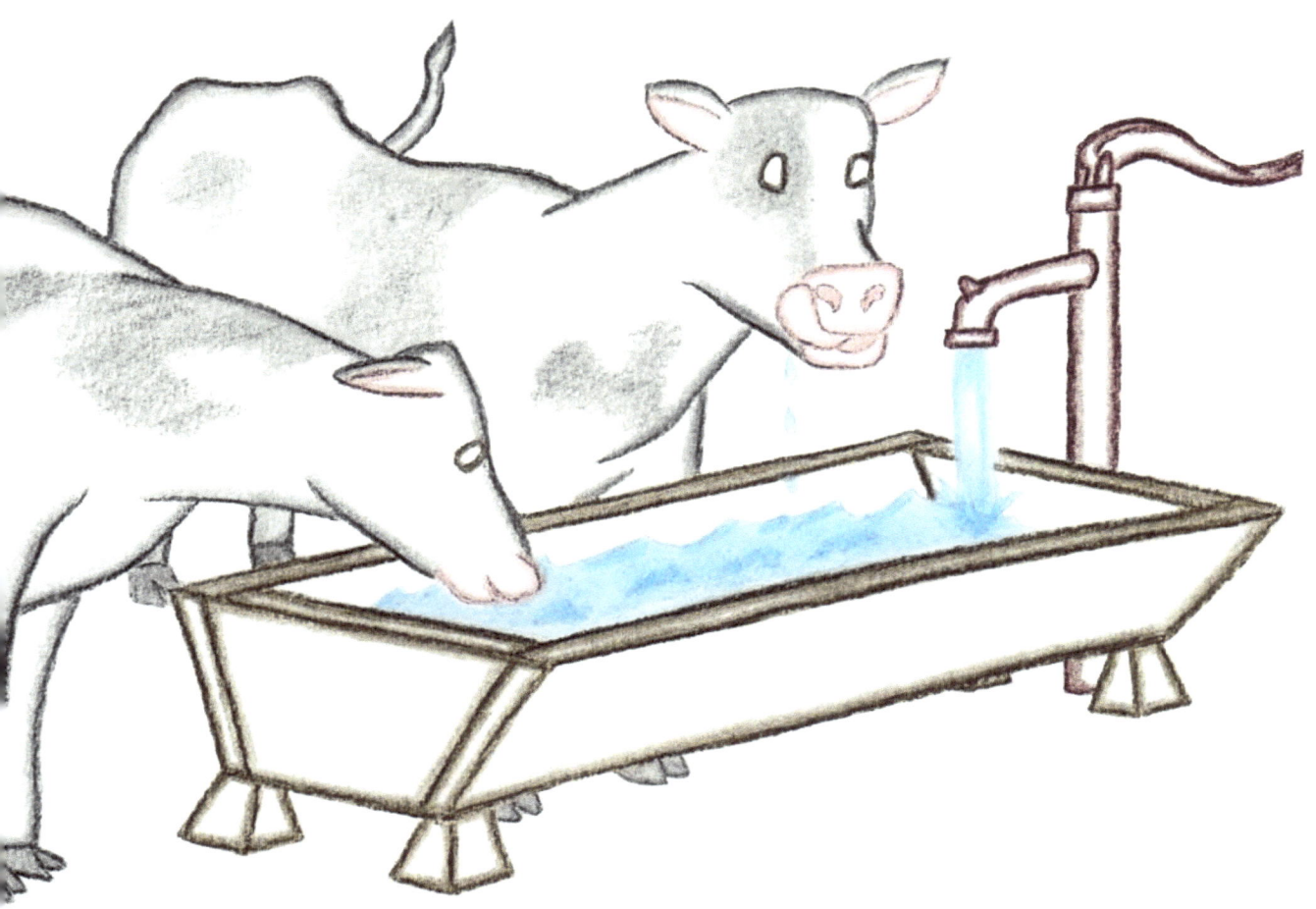

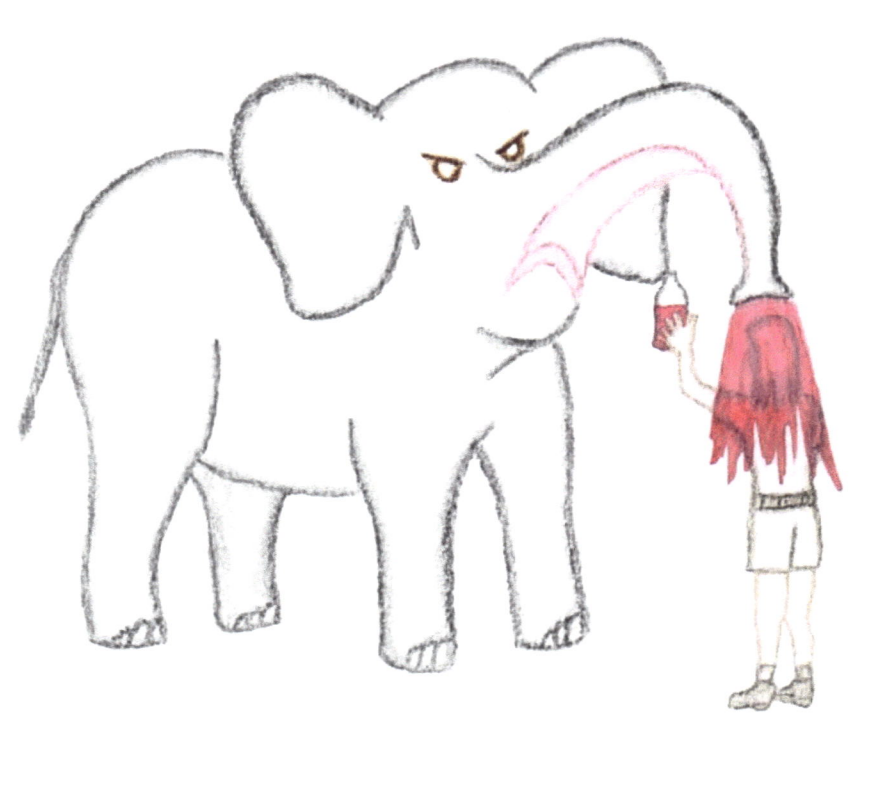

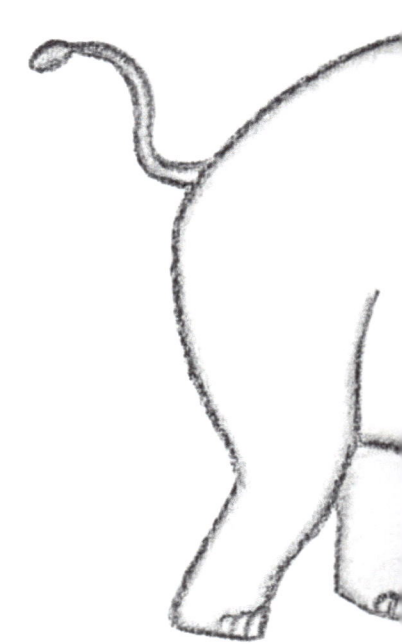

When the zookeeper feeds
the elephants lunch,
does she give them lettuce
with **syrup-filled punch?**

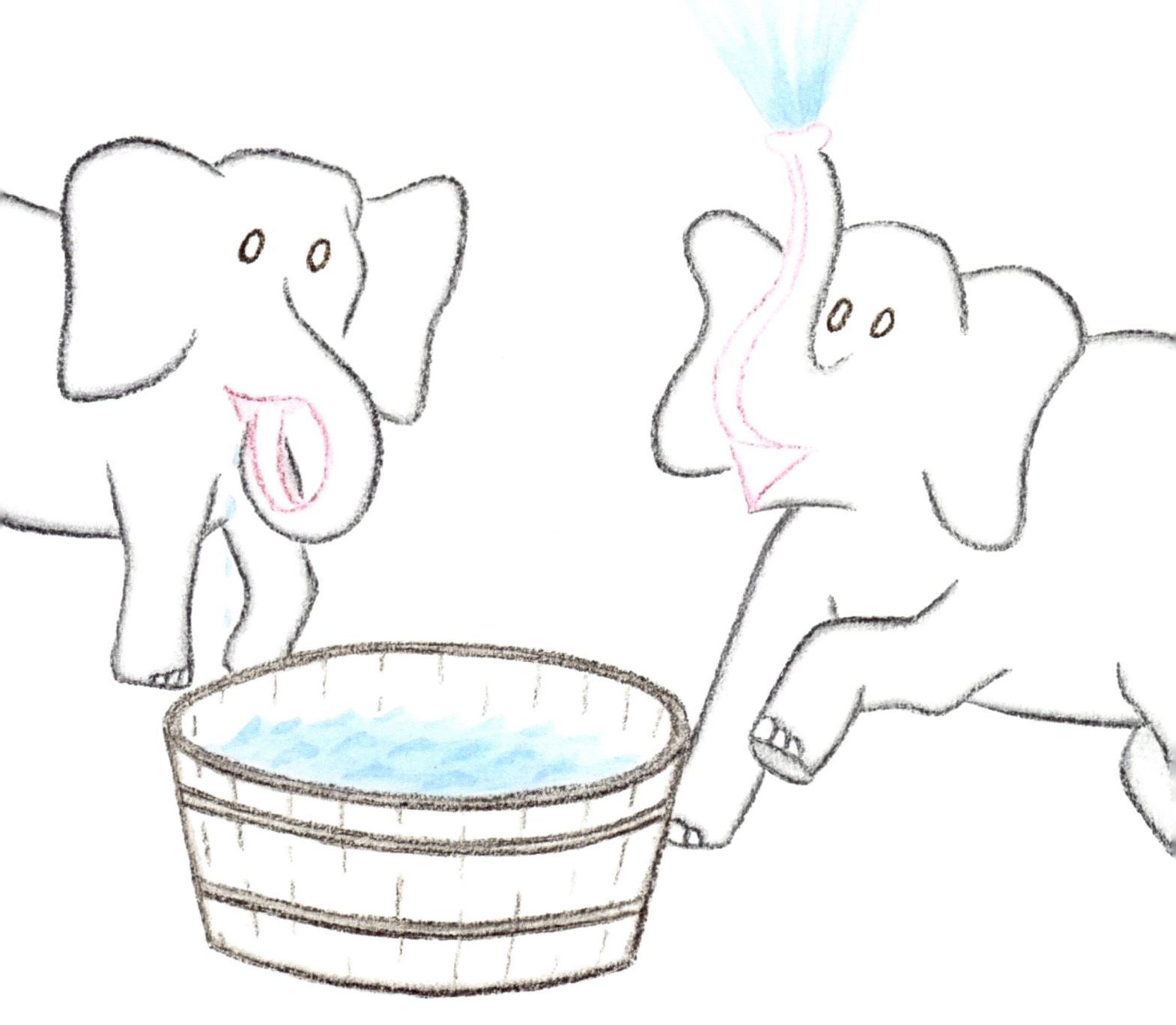

When a polar bear wants to feel really cool,

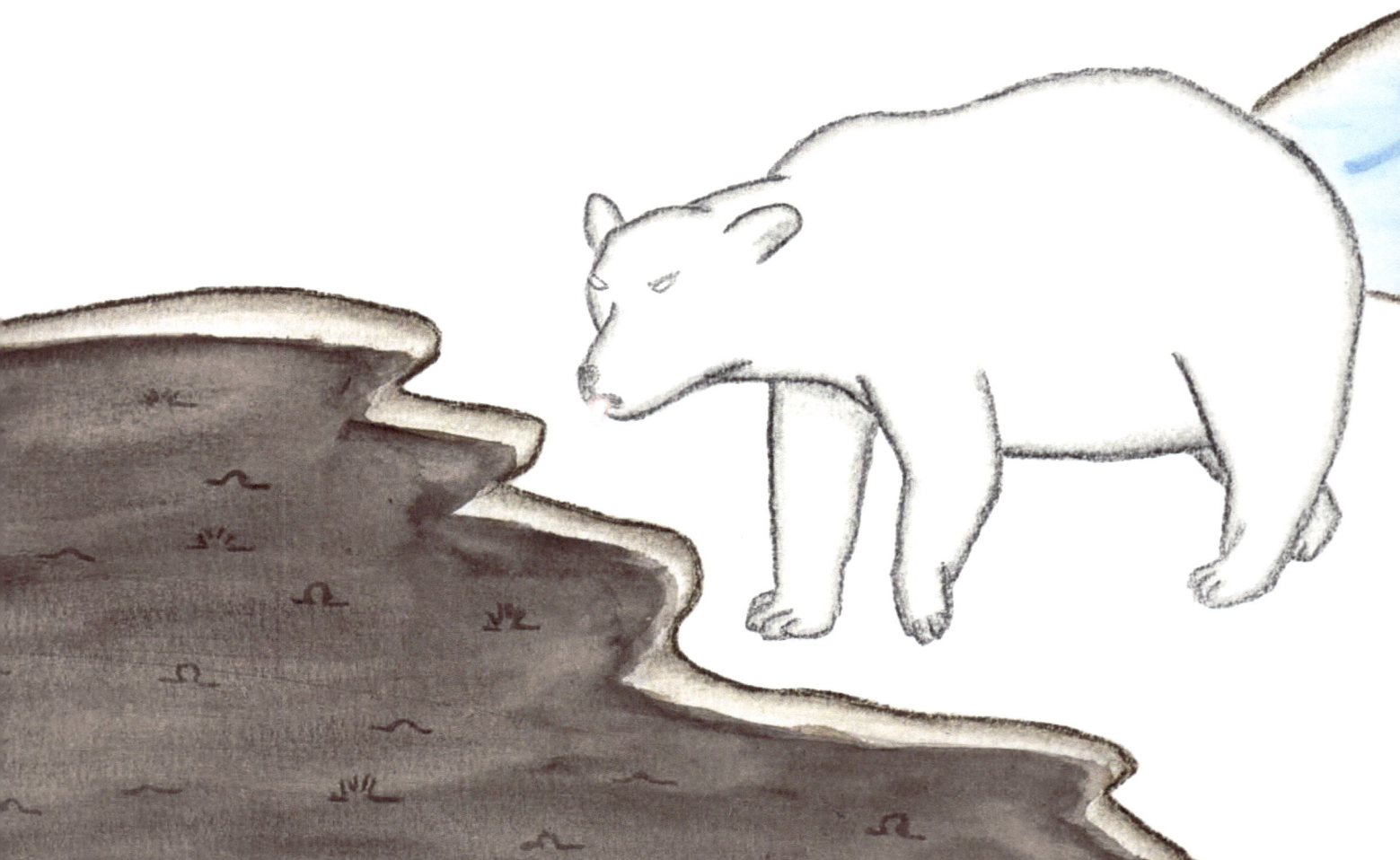

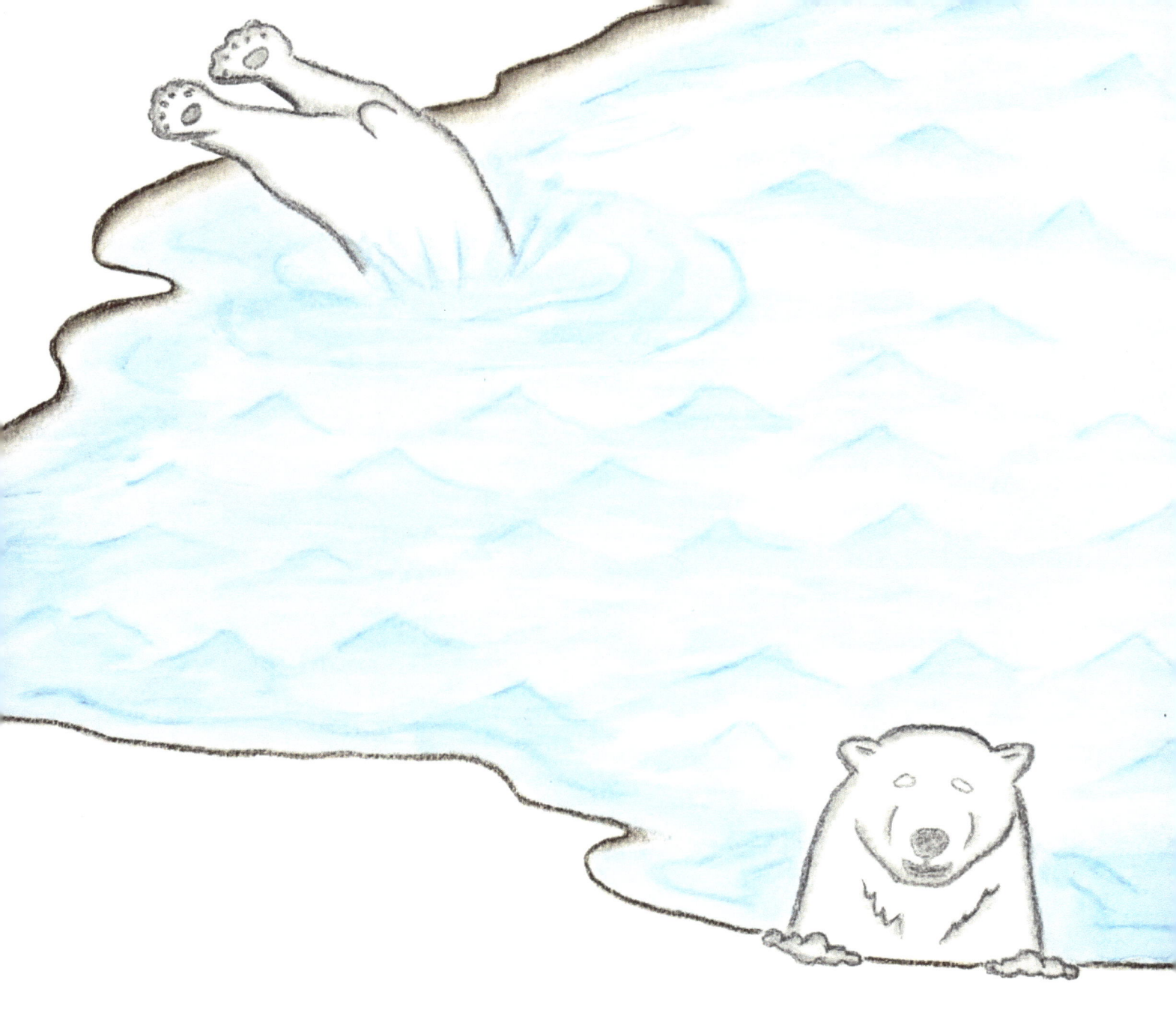

does he take a swim in a **soda pop pool?**

When the fire is raging
with fierce power,

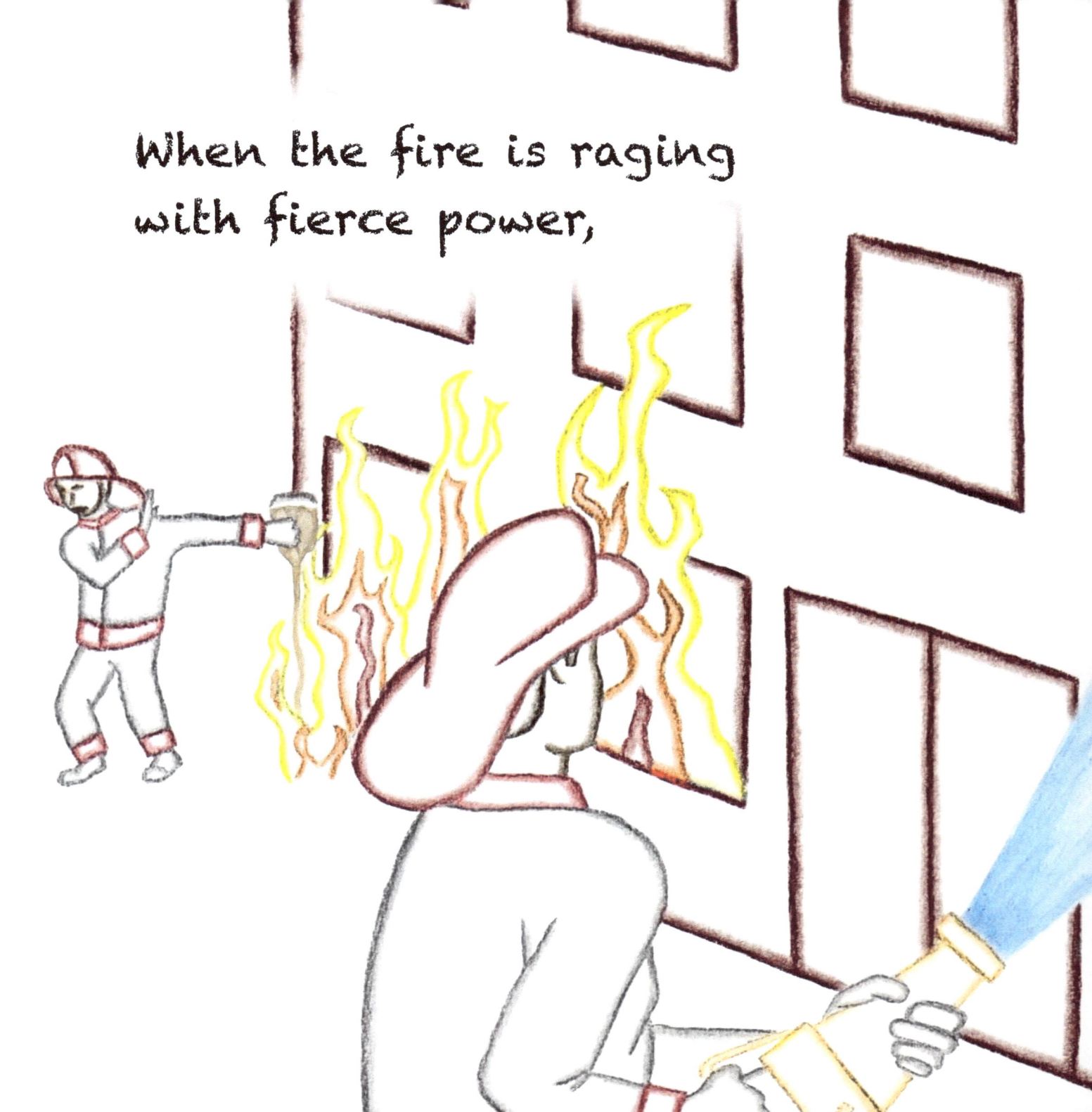

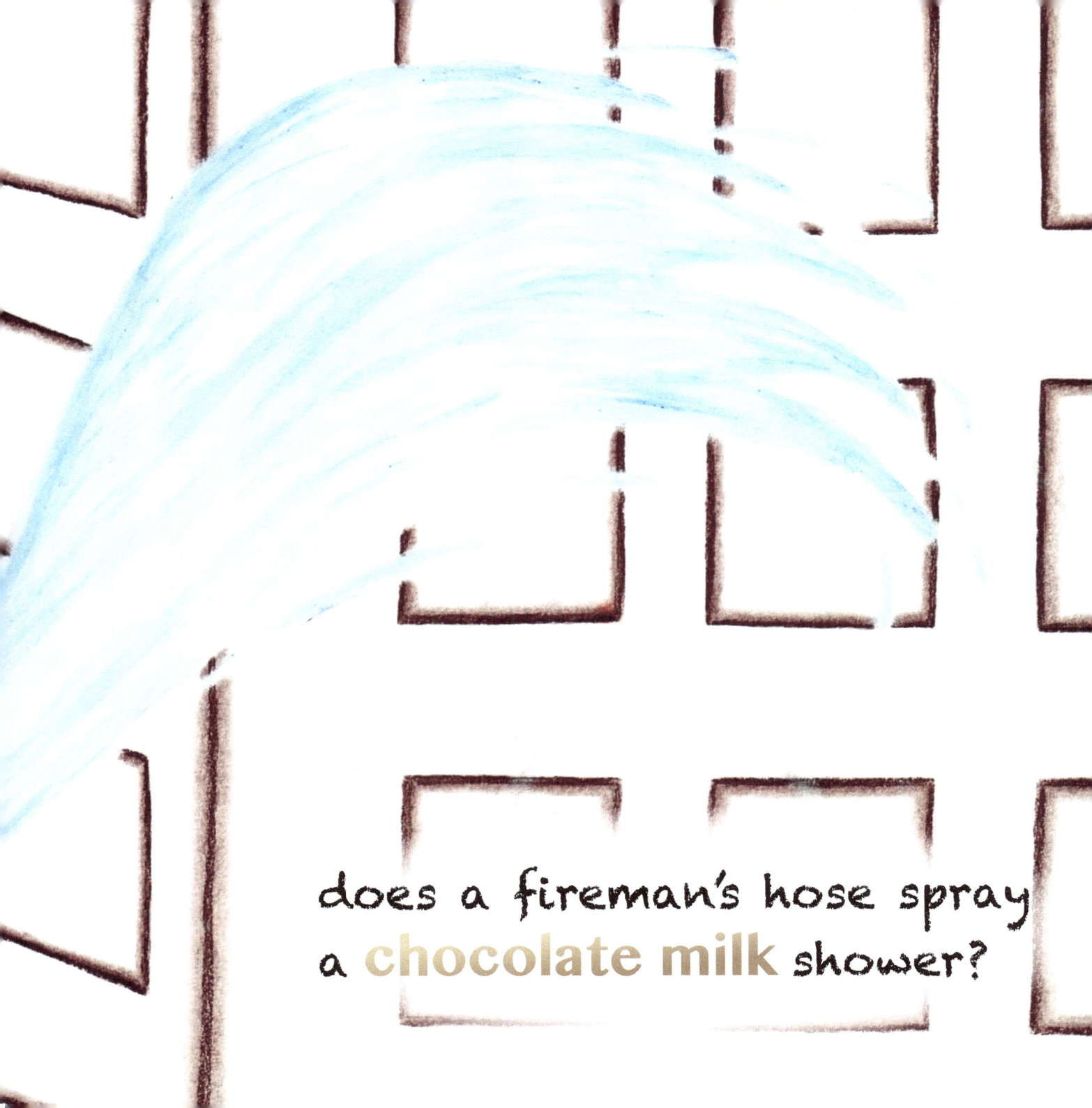

does a fireman's hose spray
a **chocolate milk** shower?

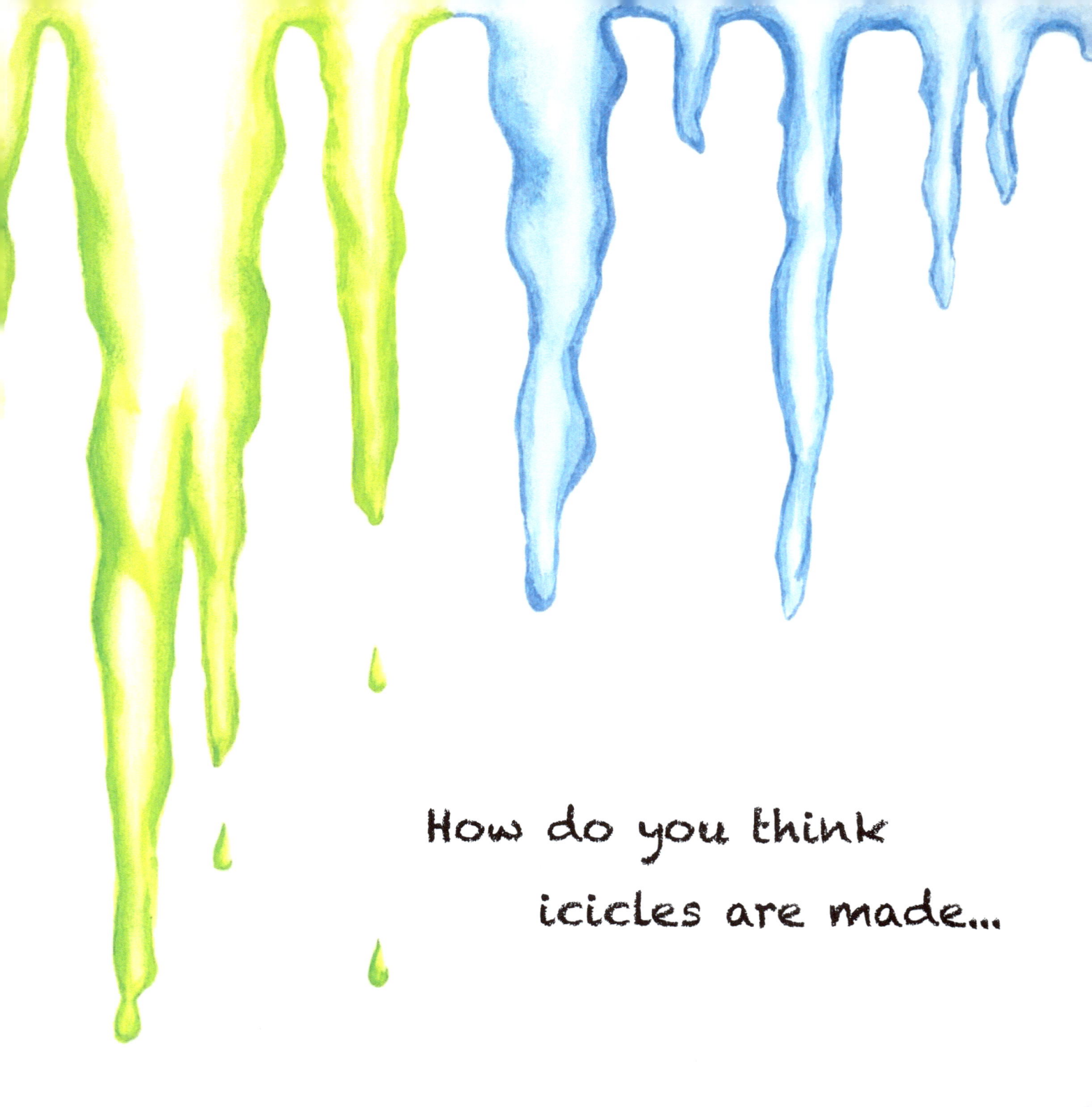

How do you think icicles are made...

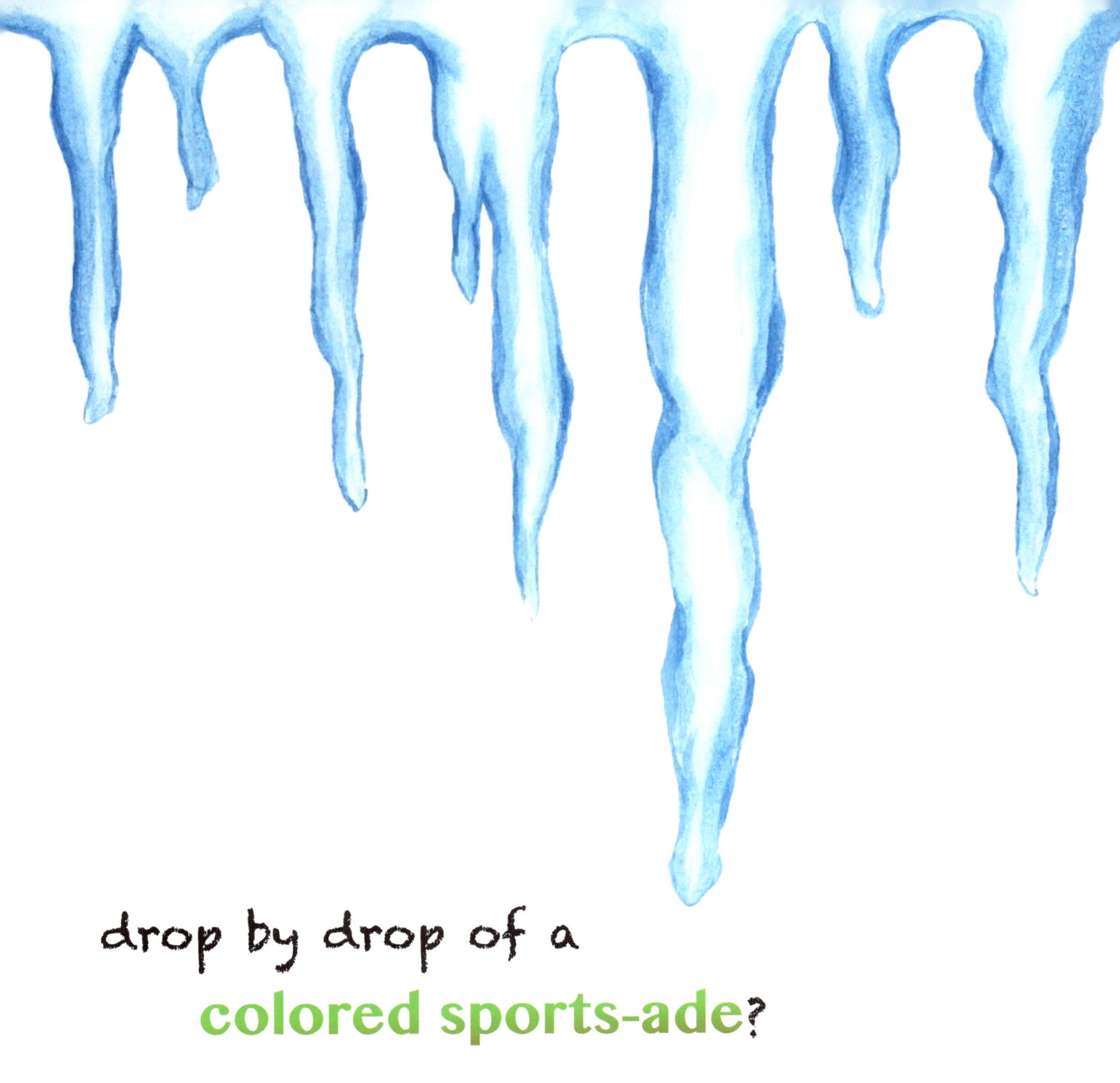

drop by drop of a

colored sports-ade?

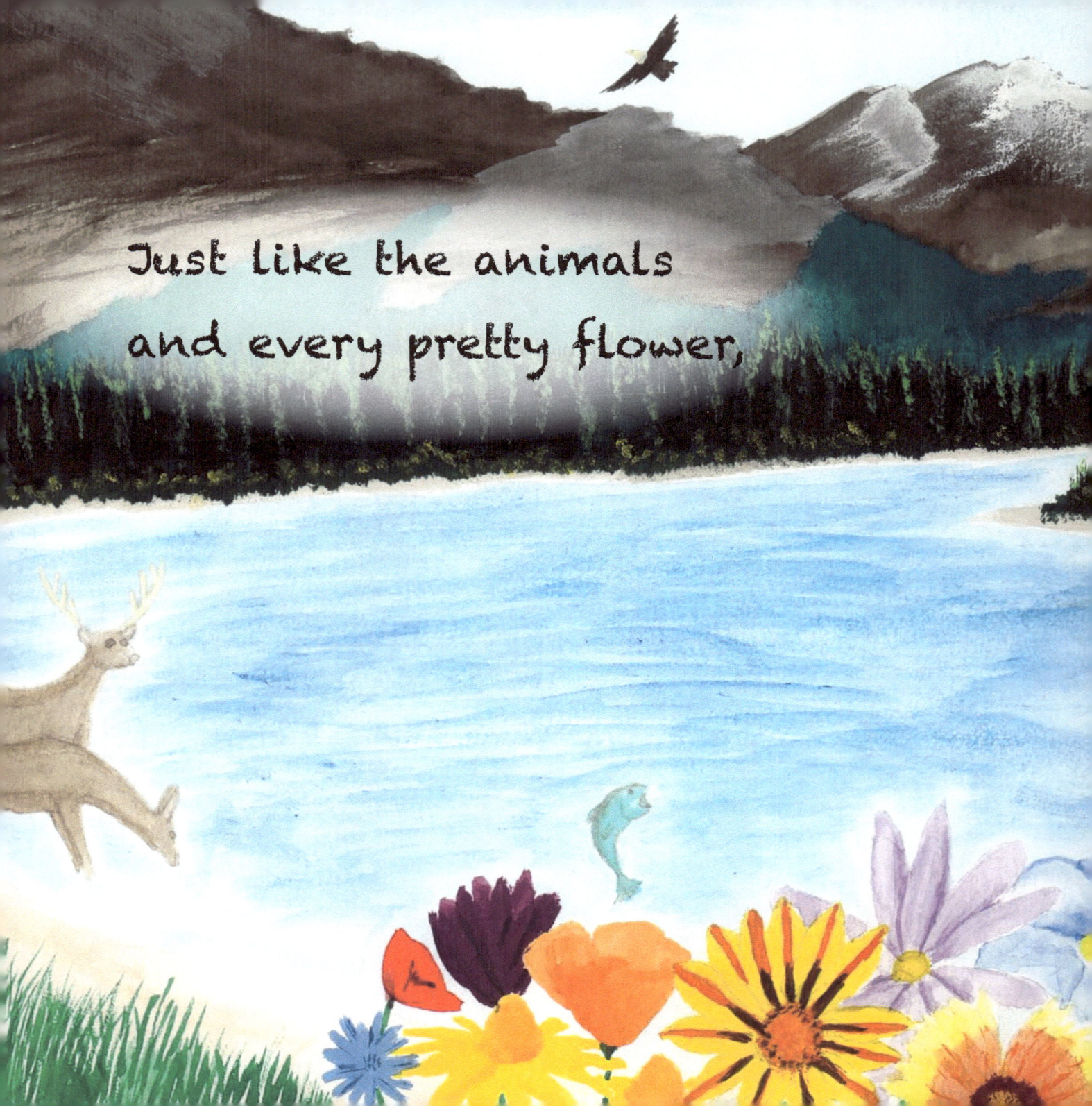

Just like the animals
and every pretty flower,

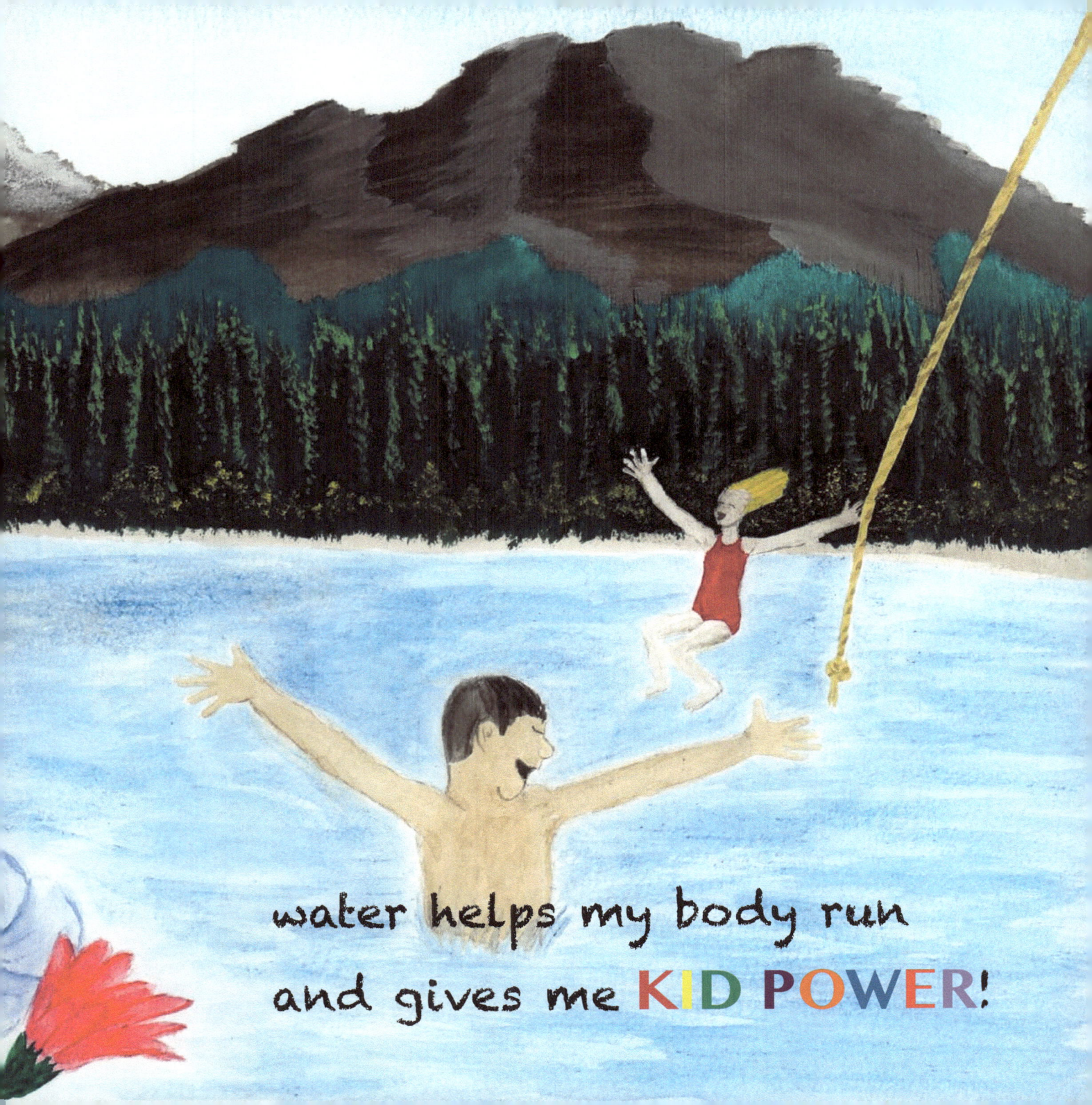

water helps my body run
and gives me KID POWER!

So when I pick up my cup
and drink it down,

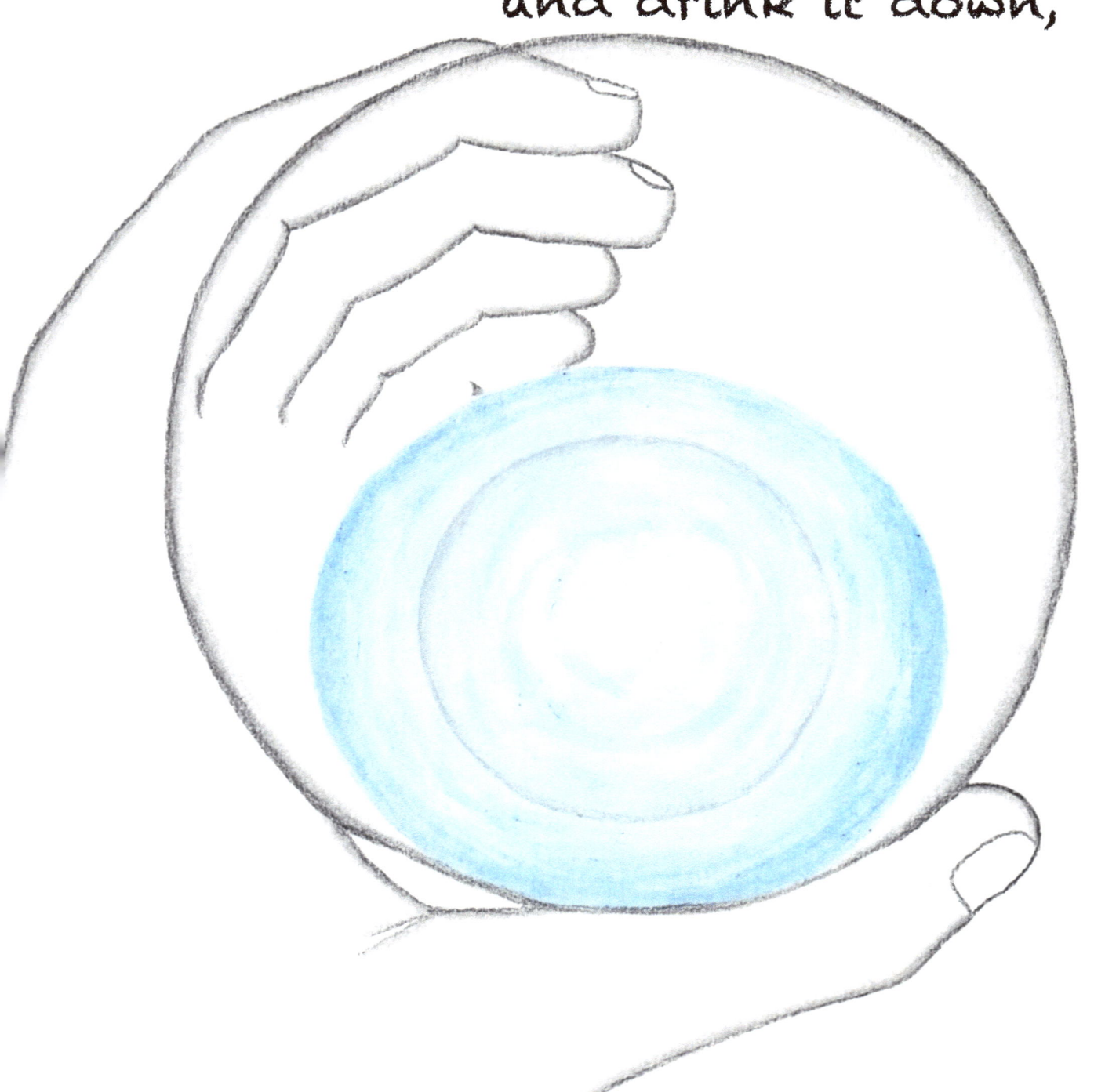

I give a cheer for water,

The Coolest Drink Around!

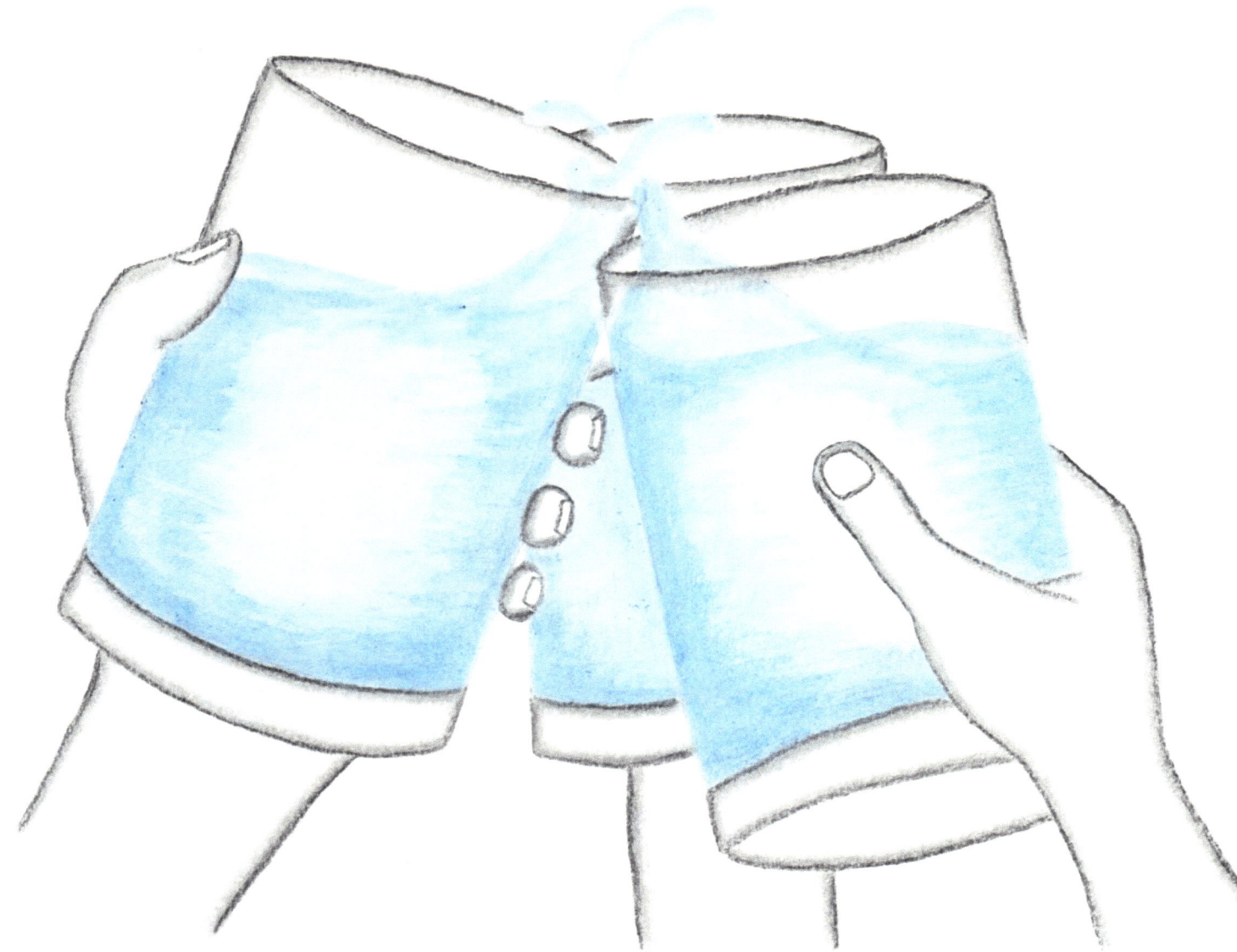

A Note to Parents

In Kenya, the quest for water dominates daily life. In fact, many women walk more than five hours a day to get clean drinking water for their families. In the United States, we have many options to obtain clean drinking water, yet many people are still thirsting and don't even realize it.

Although we don't have to walk hours to obtain clean water, we do have to do more than simply turn on the faucet. It is important to provide quality filtered water to our children. There are many inexpensive filtration options for families including Reverse Osmosis.

For more information about the current condition of our water supply and proper hydration practices, pick up a copy of <u>The Ten Commandments of Ultimate Health</u> by Dr. Greg Pitman, DC, DNBHE; available at Amazon.com.

Share to Donate!

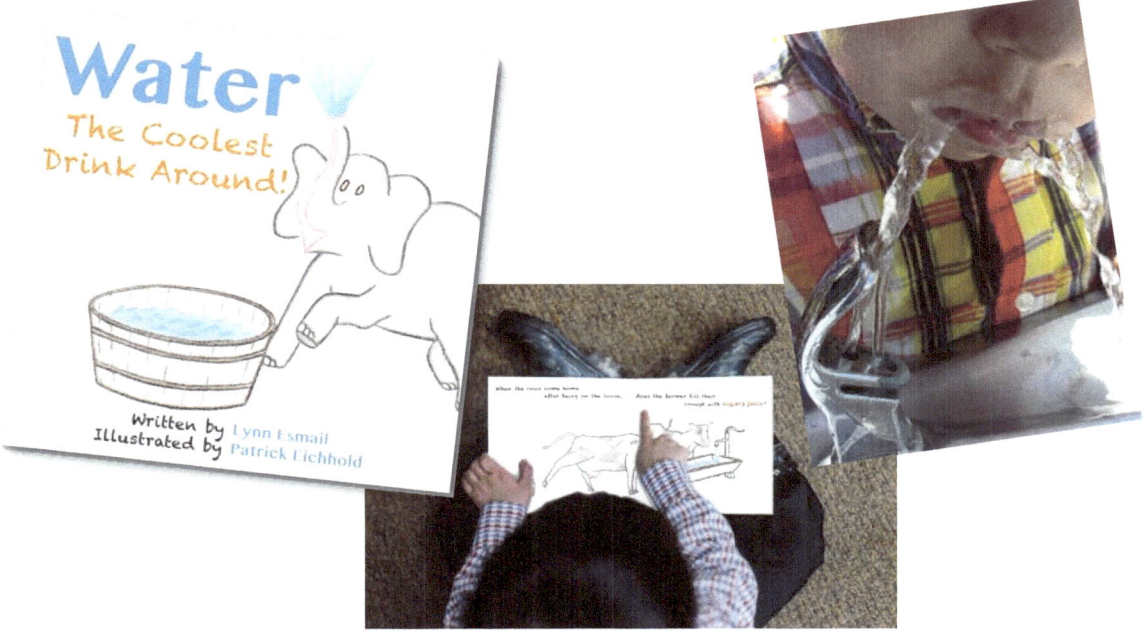

Follow us 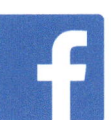   @kidbooks4health

Post pics of the book!
pics of your kids enjoying the book!
pics of your kids drinking water!

Tag your posts using #CoolestDrinkAround

When you do we'll **Donate** to Water.org

Please visit bedtimestorybooksforhealth.com for more information

About the Author

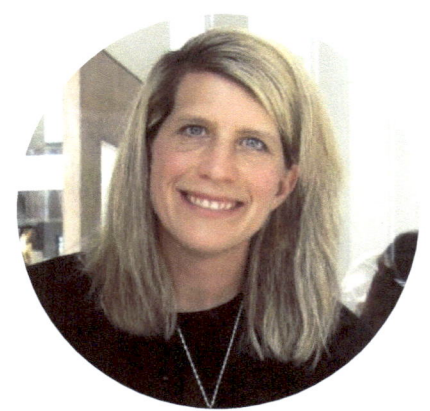

Lynn Esmail

Lynn and her husband, Jim, are the proud parents of two young boys. Lynn's journey to ultimate health began when her youngest son developed severe allergies to almost everything. When mainstream medicine offered no relief for her son's symptoms she turned to alternative methods of healing. Today her son is allergy-free! She is also the co-author of <u>The Ten Commandments of Ultimate Health</u> with Dr. Greg Pitman.

About the Illustrator

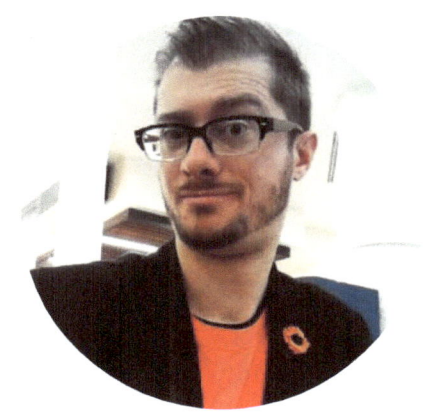

Patrick Eichhold

Patrick cannot consume enough information that will help him become the best-version-of-himself. After reading The <u>Ten Commandments of Ultimate Health</u>, he was inspired to seek out new ways of treating his depression. Through alternative medicine he not only gained relief of his symptoms of depression, but has been healed of the underlying physiological causes of his depression. Patrick is excited to explore and share more ways of experiencing true healing and ultimate health!

www.ingramcontent.com/pod-product-compliance
Lightning Source LLC
Chambersburg PA
CBHW060824290526
45792CB00005BB/1783